DRUGS
AND
MEDICINE

JENNY BRYAN

Wayland

DRUGS AND CRIME
DRUGS AND THE MEDIA
DRUGS AND MEDICINE
DRUGS AND SPORT

Designer: Helen White
Series editor: Deborah Elliott

Cover: A technician tests a new drug in a laboratory.

First published in 1992 by
Wayland (Publishers) Ltd.
61 Western Road, Hove, East Sussex BN3 1JD

British Library Cataloguing in Publication Data

Bryan, Jenny
Drugs and Medicine. – (Drugs)
I. Title II. Series
362.29

ISBN 0-7502-0316-1

Typeset by White Design
Printed by Canale C.S.p.A in Turin
Bound by AGM in France

CONTENTS

CHAPTER ONE

CURSE OR CURE ?

DO YOU take drugs? Of course you do! Whether you swallow some paracetamol for a headache, puff on a cigarette, or inject heroin into your veins, you are taking a drug. The big difference is that paracetamol will make your pain better but cigarettes, alcohol and heroin will damage your health and may even kill you.

All drugs – even paracetamol – can be harmful if they are not taken correctly. For some drugs, such as cigarettes, alcohol and heroin there is no safe dose. Knowing which drugs are safe to take and when and how to take them is vital if you, your family and your friends are to get the most from modern drugs without suffering any unwanted effects.

We have all come to expect a great deal from the drugs our doctors prescribe for us. Yet, with a few brilliant exceptions, they are not miracle cures. Nearly all of them can hurt as well as help us. We need to be able to weigh the risks against the benefits.

It is a mistake to expect a pill for every ill. Sometimes it is best to let our bodies get better on their own, without drugs. The human body has a remarkable repair system which can put right many common problems, such as coughs, colds and minor infections. However, there are times when modern drugs can be truly life-saving – as thousands of people who have suffered heart attacks, cancer or accidents will agree.

By understanding more of the science of how drugs work and how they are discovered and tested, we will be in a better position to judge whether we really want to take them.

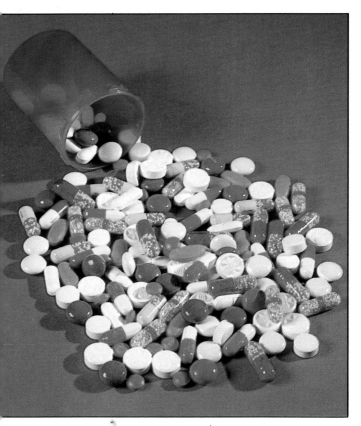

ABOVE The word drugs instils concern and fear in many people. However, we all take drugs at some point - for a stomach upset or a headache, for example.

OPPOSITE We often expect doctors to prescribe pills for every minor ache and pain. Sometimes it is better to leave our bodies to get better on their own.

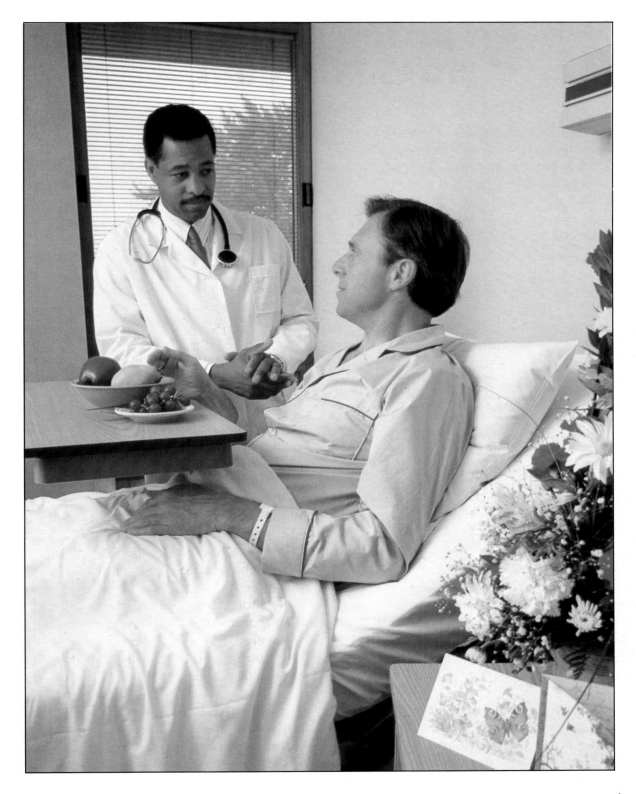

CHAPTER TWO

WHAT IS A DRUG ?

A DRUG is a substance which affects the way the body works. It can copy, increase, reduce, or block the action of one or more of the natural chemicals in the body. These chemicals are the messengers of the body; they tell our organs and other tissues what to do.

To work, natural chemicals, such as hormones and nerve transmitters, must be able to get into cells in the body. They latch on to and bind to sites on cell membranes called receptors. Each of these is tailor-made to the structure of a different chemical. Only if the chemical fits its receptor perfectly can it get into a cell - like a key unlocking a door.

In medicine, drugs can be designed to fit the same 'lock' as natural chemicals. Once on the receptor, a drug may act in the same way as the chemical it is replacing or, more often, it may block it. For example, millions of people who suffer from stomach ulcers take drugs that block receptors normally occupied by a natural chemical called histamine. The stomach needs histamine to make acid. By taking over these so called 'H2' receptors, drugs prevent histamine from working. Less acid gets into the stomach and ulcers - which form when there is too much acid - have a chance to heal.

Certain tranquillizers work in a similar way, but in the brain. They compete for receptors with natural chemicals that make us jumpy and anxious.

Some drugs work by interfering with the way our natural body chemicals are made. Many people whose blood pressure is too high are given drugs that block the action of an enzyme called ACE. This is needed to produce a chemical that makes blood vessels get narrower. By blocking ACE, doctors can make blood vessels relax and get wider, lowering the pressure of the blood flowing through them.

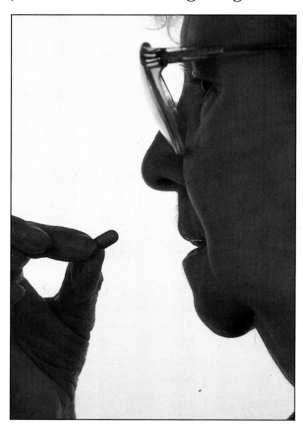

High blood pressure can sometimes be fatal. Sufferers can take drugs that block the action of ACE – the enzyme that makes blood vessels get narrower.

The false-colour X-ray of the hands of a person suffering from extreme rheumatoid arthritis. Arthritis is defined as the swelling of one or more joints, causing pain and the restriction of movement. Treatment usually involves the use of anti-inflammatory drugs, but these are of little use in severe and crippling cases.

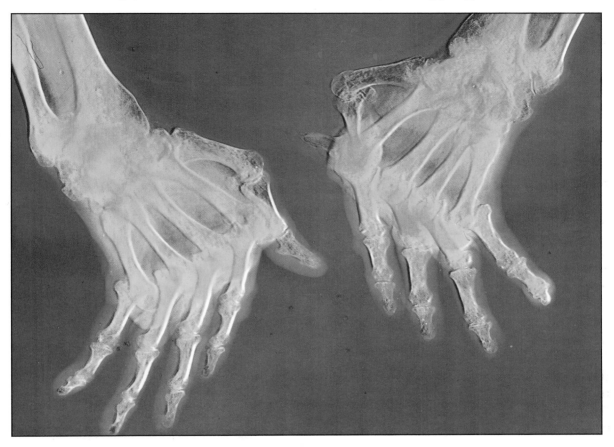

People with arthritis need drugs that block production of chemicals in the body that cause pain. These chemicals are called prostaglandins. Many painkillers block the vital enzyme which is needed for prostaglandins to be made.

You may well ask why the body should have pain chemicals in the first place! Why do we need pain? Pain is a very useful warning that something is wrong in the body. But, unfortunately, doctors cannot always treat the cause of the pain. The best they can do is treat the pain itself.

In some illnesses drugs are used to boost levels of natural chemicals that are in short supply. In these cases the drugs are made to look and act as much like the natural chemicals as possible. For example, people with diabetes do not have enough of a hormone called insulin, which is normally produced in the pancreas and is essential for the breakdown of sugar. Diabetics can now inject themselves with genetically engineered (produced by bacteria in a laboratory) human insulin.

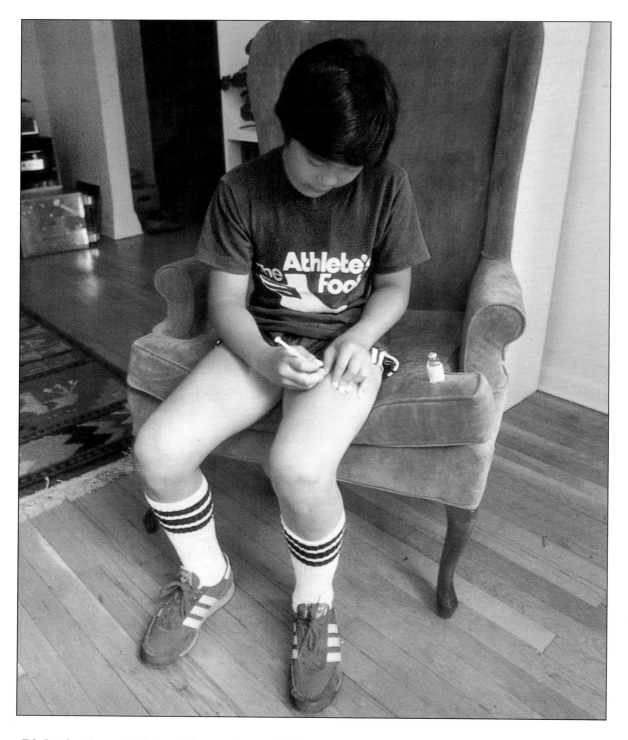

Diabetics have to inject themselves with insulin. Insulin is a protein hormone made in the pancreas that controls the amount of sugar in the blood.

Drugs are not always used to treat illnesses; they can be used to prevent them too. Vaccines are used to protect us from dozens of infections. They do this by making our bodies produce proteins called antibodies as defence against attack by micro-organisms.

Vaccines are made from some of the harmless proteins in bacteria and viruses. When they are injected into the body, the immune system responds by producing millions of antibodies. There is normally no real threat from the small quantities of the proteins used in a vaccine. But later, if the body is attacked by the whole bacterium or virus, not just its harmless proteins, the antibodies will recognize it as alien and destroy it.

Drugs can also be used to confuse the body. This is what the contraceptive pill does. By rearranging a woman's hormonal timetable each month, the pill prevents her from releasing an egg and makes her womb hostile to sperm. So no egg is fertilized and the woman does not become pregnant.

Unfortunately, drugs have unwanted as well as useful effects. If a drug works in one part of the body it is almost certain that it will work in other parts too.

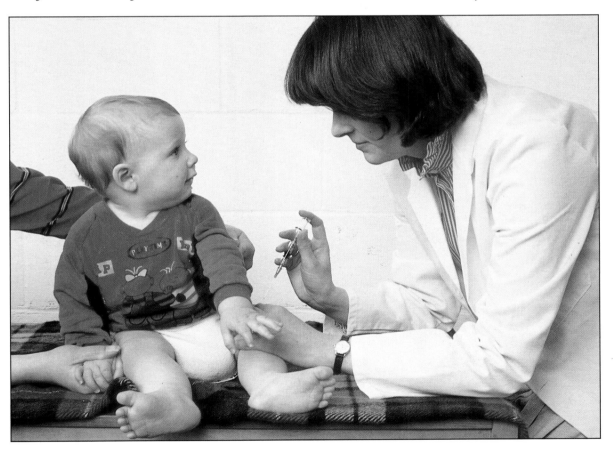

Young babies are given a series of innoculations (injections) against diptheria, polio and whooping cough by the time they are six months old.

A packet of oral contraceptives for a method of birth control known as 'the pill'. The pill consists of one or more synthetic female sex hormones which prevent ovulation.

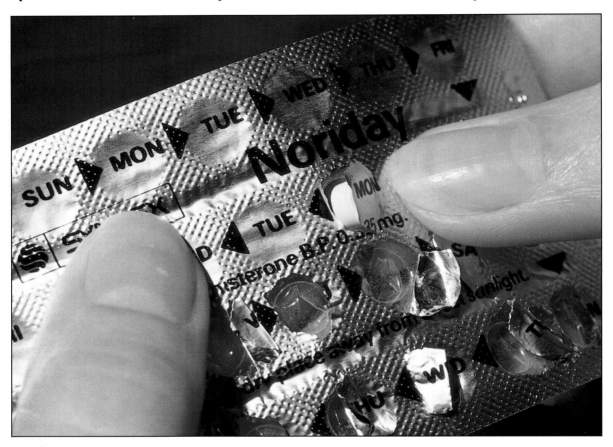

Receptor sites may look the same in two very different parts of the body. It can be dangerous if a drug works in a place where it is not wanted. For example, heart and lung tissue both contain beta receptors. These help to control the width of blood vessels and airways and the rate at which the heart beats.

People with high blood pressure or an abnormal heart rate may be given drugs that block the beta receptors in their hearts and blood vessels. If their breathing is normal it will not matter much if some of the beta receptors in their lungs are blocked too. However, if they have breathing problems, such as asthma, it could be dangerous to block beta receptors in their lungs. So, if possible, people with high blood pressure and asthma should not take drugs that block beta receptors.

The mind can also affect how drugs work. If an inactive, dummy pill is given to 100 people, it will work in about thirty cases. The more that people believe in a treatment the more likely they are to feel better - and nobody knows why. Whatever the reason, it is important always to take account of this so called 'placebo' effect in judging whether a drug really works.

CHAPTER THREE

WHERE DO DRUGS GO ?

IT TAKES at least fifteen minutes for a drug to go from the mouth down into the stomach and intestine, get into the bloodstream, travel to the place it is needed and start working. Compare that with the few seconds it takes for an anaesthetic to work when it is injected straight into a vein.

Drugs would definitely work much more quickly if they did not have to go through the stomach and intestine. Some drugs, such as insulin, have to be injected because they would be destroyed by the digestive juices if they went through the intestine.

No one likes injections so, unless a treatment needs to work immediately or it cannot be put into tablet form, doctors normally prescribe drugs that can be taken by mouth. First stop will be the stomach. Here, a solid tablet will start to break down into small particles, ready to move on to the small intestine. A drug which is already in liquid form will pass through more quickly. Particles of drug move across the wall of the intestine into tiny blood vessels which carry blood through to the liver.

Many things can affect how quickly drugs are absorbed from the gut. They tend to be absorbed more quickly when taken with food, for example, because the transport systems are already switched on.

What happens in the liver will depend on the type of drug. Some drugs are broken down in the liver and only a small amount gets back into the bloodstream.

Drug companies must allow for this when deciding how much to put in each tablet.

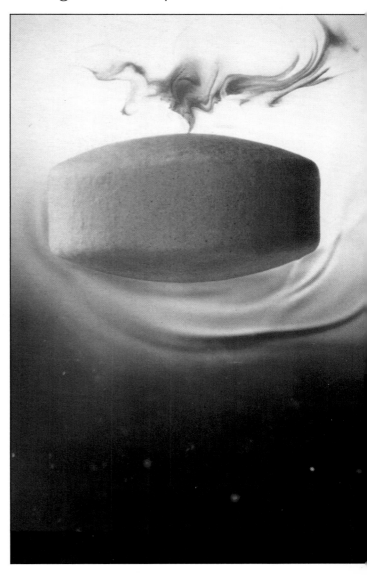

This abstract image shows the sustained release of a drug from a tablet.

11

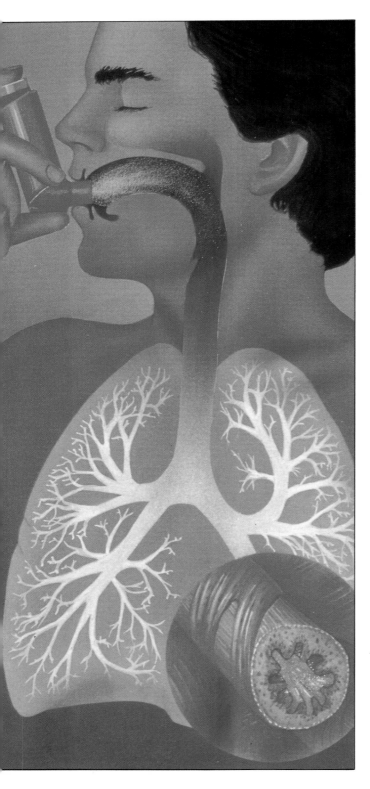

Other drugs pass through the liver untouched. The liver is the last big hurdle for a drug. Once it is back in the bloodstream it can go at last to the place where it is meant to work, though organs which have the biggest blood supply, such as the heart, kidneys and brain for example, will take priority.

A drug that is to go deep into brain tissue must have special properties. This is because it is much harder for things to get out of blood vessels into brain cells than in other parts of the body. Any drug that does not manage to get into cells in the body will eventually pass through the kidneys and be excreted (passed out) in the urine.

Some drugs are given in an inactive form. They only become active when they come into contact with chemicals present in the body.

Over the years, drug companies have developed clever ways of controlling the speed with which drugs are released into cells and how long they stay in the body before they are excreted.

It would be dangerous if all the contents of a drug were released at once. Someone with high blood pressure, for example, needs a drug that will lower the pressure slowly and smoothly, not all at once – or they would pass out!

A cutaway drawing showing the use of a Ventolin inhaler to control asthma. The inhaler contains a drug called salbutamol which makes the bronchial muscles widen, thereby allowing air to pass to the lungs. Bronchial asthma is caused by the narrowing of the airways – a result of the lining surfaces swelling and an increase in the production of mucous.

A close-up of low-power, red argon laser beams being directed through four fibre optic waveguides to treat a cancer tumour. The beams activate a drug previously injected into the patient. This drug does not affect normal cells, but is absorbed by cancerous cells.

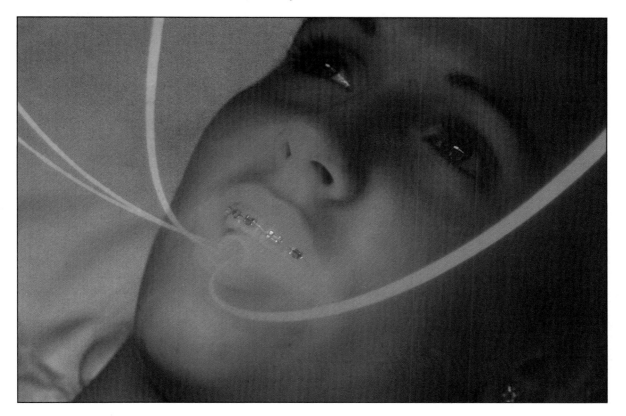

People with long-term illnesses, such as arthritis, need painkilling drugs to work for as long as possible. This is why many drugs are designed to work for a full twenty-four hours. Within a single tablet or capsule, minute particles of the drug can be wrapped inside coatings of different thicknesses or with different chemical properties so that they are released at different times.

Some layers will be released straight-away, others take hours after the drug enters the body. The result is a drug that works for many hours. Some drugs work for months! Women who suffer from menopausal symptoms, such as hot flushes, because the levels of some of their hormones have gone down, can have a drug implant put under their skin. This releases replacement hormones for several months. So there is no need to take tablets every day.

Other drugs can be taken through the skin. They are put into a sticking plaster on the skin which gradually releases the drug over a period of several days.

People with lung problems, such as asthma, want instant relief when they are wheezy. They do not want to wait for a drug to go through their intestine or even their skin before it reaches their lungs.

A cancer patient being prepared for radiotherapy treatment.

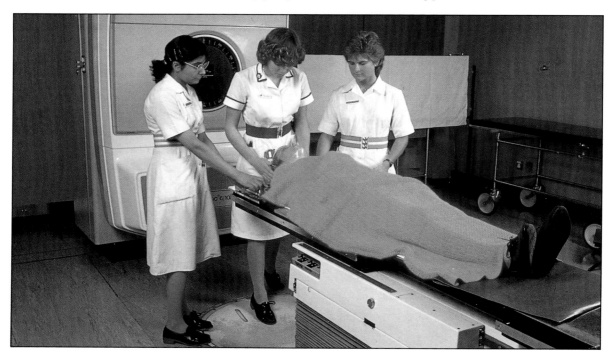

They inhale drugs straight into their lungs. They can feel better in seconds.

In the future doctors hope to target drugs much more accurately to different parts of the body. This should help reduce side effects. For example, at present anti-cancer drugs often cause serious side effects because they kill normal cells as well as tumour cells. Scientists are currently experimenting with many different ways of getting future anti-cancer drugs to 'home in' on tumour cells alone, leaving healthy cells untouched.

Some of the research has been going on for quite a while. Doctors are already using anti-cancer drugs with antibodies 'tagged' on to their surfaces. The antibodies are made to recognize proteins on the surface of cancer cells which are not found on normal, healthy cells. This means that the drugs attack only the cancer cells and leave all the normal cells alone.

The same method is used to target radioactive agents to tumour cells. Radioactive chemicals are 'tagged' with antibodies which carry them to tumour cells where they release their lethal radiation.

Another method uses light or heat to 'switch on' anti-cancer drugs. These are swallowed in their inactive state. Light or heat is then applied to the part of the body with the cancer. This activates the anti-cancer drug as it is passes through the tumour cells. The drug remains inactive in the rest of the body and does not causes any damage.

Hopefully, scientists will perfect better ways of getting drugs to the places they are needed most and will thus reduce the risk of unwanted side effects.

CHAPTER FOUR

GOOD DRUGS AND BAD DRUGS

THE most successful prescription drug of the last few years has been for one stomach ulcers. The reason it is so successful is that it is very effective and it has few side effects. It has also withstood the test of time. It has fought off the challenge of newer, rival drugs which are probably just as good – and may be even better –

because doctors are more familiar with it. They know that millions of people around the world have taken it and, after several years, there appear to be no terrible hidden dangers.

Newer drugs may be just as safe but they have not been used by as many people, for so long. They simply cannot

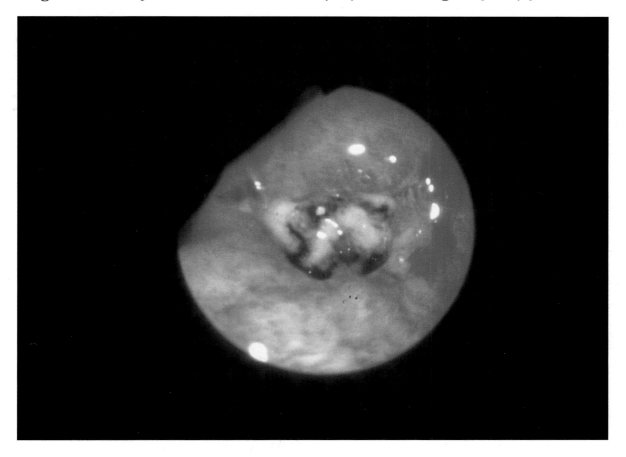

An endoscope image of a stomach ulcer – a disruption of the stomach lining caused by acid and bile. Symptoms include vomiting and severe stomach pains after eating. The causes are related to diet, alcohol, stress and certain drugs.

15

boast the same impressive track record.

When a drug company starts looking for a bestselling drug it has two main options. It can try to find a drug to cure a disease for which there is no really effective treatment. Or it can make a drug which is similar to something already available but will have important advantages; it is more effective, is easier to take or has fewer side effects.

In the first group would go new drugs for cancer, nerve disorders, such as multiple sclerosis, or psychiatric conditions, such as schizophrenia. Diseases which already have quite effective treatment include high blood pressure, minor infections and asthma.

Companies will make most money from a drug that is a major advance on current treatment. However, this type of research also carries the greatest risk. It will cost more, take longer and all efforts may be wasted if a suitable drug is not found.

Not only must the drug be safe and effective it must be relatively easy to make and, in most cases, it must be possible to produce it as a tablet or capsule. Patients do not want to inject themselves several times a day unless the drug is a life-saver and cannot be taken by mouth.

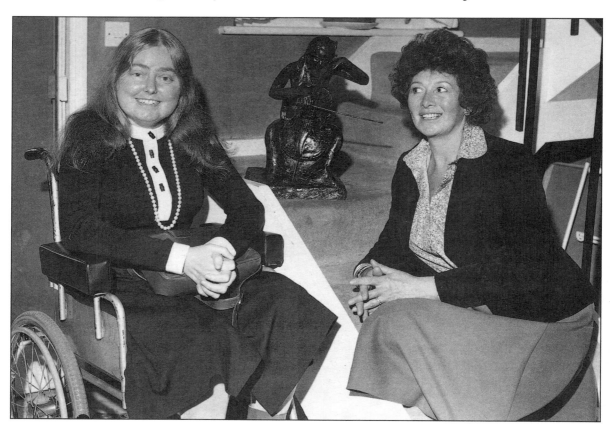

The world famous celloist Jacqueline Dupre (left) had multiple sclerosis. There is no cure as yet for this debilitating disease which affects the central nervous system and can lead to speech and sight disorders and partial paralysis.

Bad drugs that have too many side effects or are too difficult to take are discarded as soon as possible. However, sometimes drug companies spend a fortune on research before discovering that a drug is no good. It may even get on to the market before doctors realize it is unsafe or does not work well enough.

There is much less risk in looking for a drug which is similar to other drugs already on the market. As long as there are not too many rivals, there can still be a lot of money to be made if the drug is for a condition that is very common, such as heart disease, arthritis or asthma.

There is however, growing pressure on drug companies to prove that their new drugs are significantly better than those already available.

RISKS AND BENEFITS

If you take a drug you need to be sure that the benefits to your health are worth the side effects. Drugs may not always be the best solution.

All drugs have some side effects, but these should be as mild and rare as possible. When you have a cold you may take something to ease your throat and lower your temperature. But if the drug

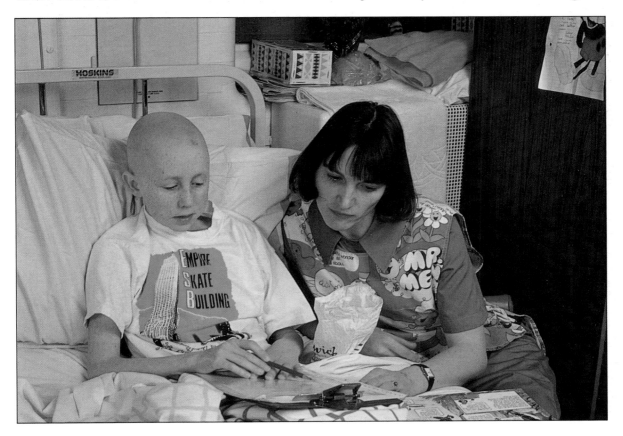

This boy has leukaemia, a type of cancer in which the bone marrow and other blood-forming organs produce large numbers of abnormal white blood cells. Chemotherapy, used to treat the disease, causes hair loss and nausea.

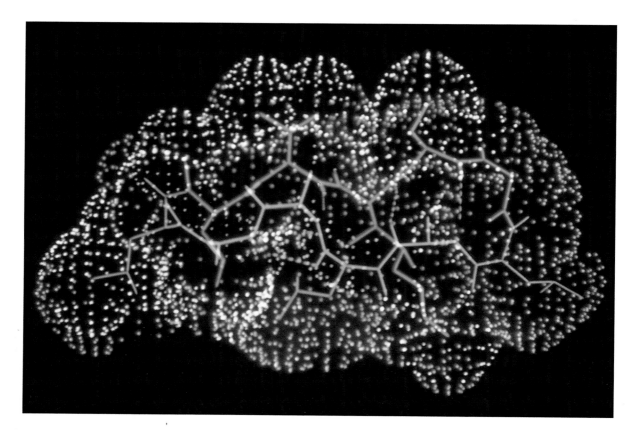

A computer graphics image of a cyclosporin molecule. Cyclosporin-A is given to organ transplant patients to reduce the risk of tissue rejection.

made you feel sick you probably would not want to take it. After all, a cold will get better on its own.

One in ten children suffer from asthma. Many take drugs to reduce the inflammation in their lungs so they do not get wheezy. There is a small risk that if they take one of these drugs they will sometimes sound a bit hoarse and croaky. But most will probably feel this is a small price to pay to be able to play soccer, tennis and other sports.

Some people have to inject themselves every day with insulin because they are diabetic. Injections are not very nice but without insulin they would become very ill. Again, the discomfort is a small price to pay for good health.

Each year a small number of children are diagnosed with leukaemia – a cancer of the blood. The treatment is unpleasant but without it the patients would probably die. The drugs they must take will make them feel sick, their hair will fall out and they may get nasty infections. But the drugs may well cure their cancer.

To decide whether the benefits of drugs are worth the risks, we first need to know what the drugs are. Doctors should be able to explain what drugs will do, whether they are likely to work and what are the side effects. Are those side effects mild or severe, common or rare?

Many drugs now have leaflets to accompany them which answer some of these questions and it is well worth reading them. But if you or someone you know is worried about the drugs they are taking they should be sure to ask a doctor or pharmacist about them.

We cannot expect to understand as much about drugs as doctors. But we should be prepared to take some responsibility for our health. With the right information we can take part in the decisions about our treatment – such as whether the likely benefits are worth the possible risks.

LIFE–SAVING DRUGS

Aspirin, penicillin, beta blockers, H2 antagonists, corticosteroids, cyclosporin, clotbusters. Each of these drugs or group of drugs was an important medical breakthrough in its day.

Some, such as aspirin, continue to surprise us. It is only in the last few years that doctors have realized that aspirin, which has been used in one form or another for centuries to relieve pain, can prevent strokes and heart attacks.

Other drugs, like penicillin, were not only important breakthroughs in their own right but led the way to other advances.

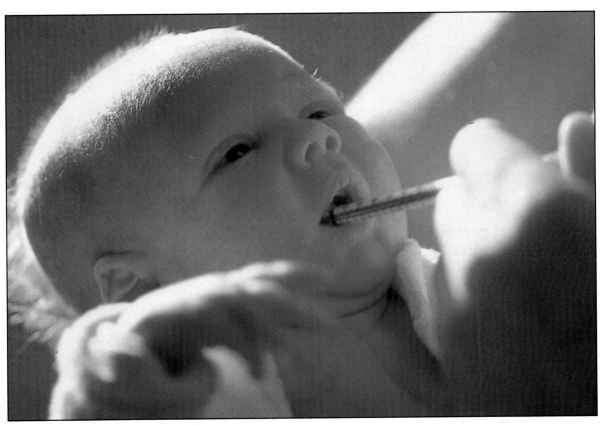

This baby is being given Cyclosporin-A through a syringe following his heart transplant operation. It is believed that babies are less likely to reject transplanted organs than adults because of their younger, less active immune systems.

19

A false-colour coronary aniogram (X-ray) of a heart. Coronary aniography is used to work out the extent of heart disease.

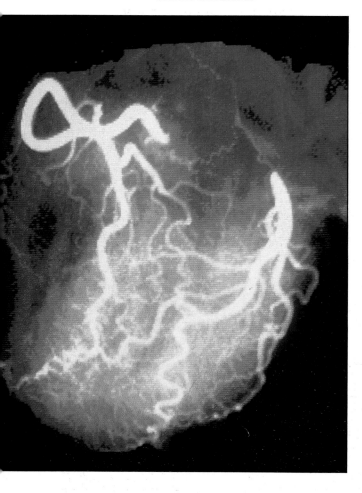

Since penicillin was discovered in 1928, dozens of new antibiotics have been developed to fight bacterial infection. As bacteria have learned how to beat some of those antibiotics, scientists have been able to make new drugs to continue the fight against infection.

Infections, such as tuberculosis, bronchitis and pneumonia, which used to wipe out whole families can now be treated effectively with antibiotics.

Beta blockers have been used to treat high blood pressure since the early 1960s. They remain the first choice of drugs for the treatment of this common condition. Not only do they keep blood pressure under control, they help prevent people who have had a heart attack from having a further attack.

Until H2 antagonists became available in the mid 1970s, people with stomach ulcers had surgery to cut the nerves to their stomach so that acid was no longer released. Within a few years that operation was history!

In the last forty years corticosteroids have revolutionized the treatment of many conditions where there is inflammation. These include asthma, eczema and arthritis. They are also used in transplant surgery to prevent the rejection of donated organs.

Without cyclosporin, kidney and heart transplants would never have become the almost routine operations they are today. Surgeons had perfected their technical skills but until cyclosporin was used in the early 1980s many operations failed because of rejection problems.

Clotbusters became news in the late 1980s when doctors discovered that if people were given them within a few hours of a heart attack they were more likely to survive. The drugs dissolve blood clots that block arteries to the heart, thus giving it a greater chance of getting better.

It will be a few years yet before we know if clotbusters will have the same impact on medicine as their revolutionary predecessors. They have a lot to live up to!

USEFUL DRUGS

A drug does not have to be a life-saver to be a useful advance in medical treatment.

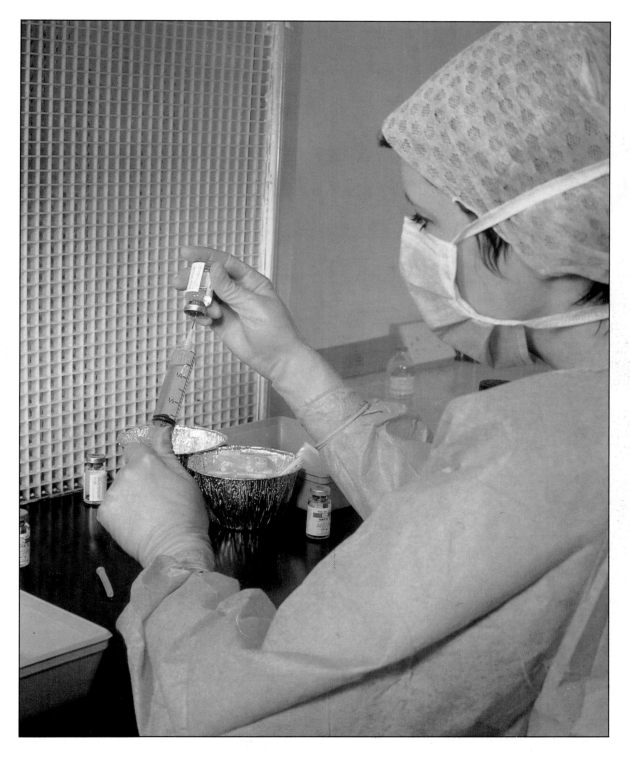

A pharmacist prepares a drug in a hospital clean room.

A positron emission tomography (PET) scan of the human brain showing evidence of Alzheimer's disease. Symptoms are loss of memory, dementia and slow death.

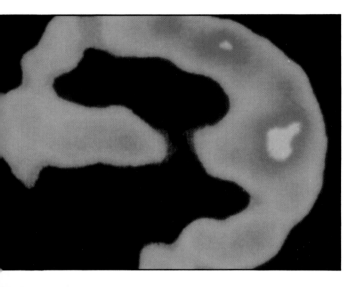

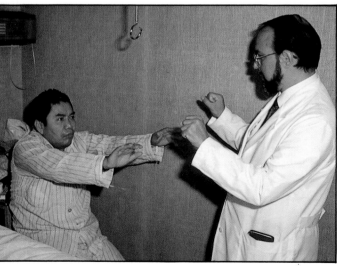

A doctor examines a man suffering from Parkinson's disease in a hospital in Mexico. People who suffer from Parkinson's disease have great difficulty in controlling their movement.

Now that so many potentially fatal diseases have been brought under control, drugs are needed that will improve the way we live as well as helping us to live much longer.

Effective vaccines mean that far fewer children growing up today know the misery of measles, mumps, diptheria or whooping cough. It is only by continuing to vaccinate large numbers of children that we can hope to keep these infections under control.

Young asthmatics can lead full, active lives thanks not only to drugs that help prevent asthma attacks but also to others that relieve symptoms in seconds when they do occur. These drugs – bronchodilators – make the airways in the lungs relax, so more air can get in and out.

Many young people with eczema can avoid the distressing, itchy rashes that their parents and grandparents suffered by rubbing effective anti-inflammatory drugs on to affected skin.

Young women can grow up safe from the worry of unwanted children, thanks to the contraceptive pill, though this does not, of course, protect them from the threat of AIDS. Also, for the one in eight couples who find it difficult to get pregnant, there are many drugs that can help restore hormone levels and improve the chances of conceiving.

Middle-aged women no longer need to be plagued by menopausal symptoms, or worry that their bones will become thin and brittle as they get older. Hormone replacement therapy (HRT) can restore the natural balance of female hormones and even protect older women from suffering heart disease.

Now that we can all expect to live longer we do not want to live our last ten

A tiny example of the many thousands of drugs available to doctors for prescriptions.

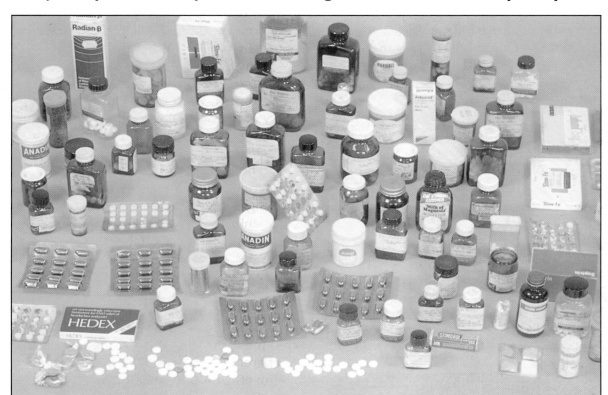

or twenty years disabled by diseases such as arthritis, heart disease, strokes or dementia. Some advances have already been made. A number of drugs can relieve the pain and stiffness of arthritis and even treat the inflammation that causes it. However, effective drugs are still needed.

By controlling blood pressure, doctors can reduce the risk of older people getting heart attacks or strokes. Some progress has also been made in treating nerve disorders such as Parkinson's disease – a condition in which older people gradually lose control over their movements and speech and sometimes their thoughts.

There is still a long way to go in finding drugs that will stop or, better still, reverse the mental problems which occur in

dementia. This will be one of the many great challenges for scientists of the twenty-first century.

'ME-TOOS'

There are about 4000 drugs available to doctors for prescriptions in Britain. Very few of these are life-savers or useful advances. Most are 'me-toos'. They were developed deliberately to copy successful drugs already on the market.

Chemically, they have to be slightly different. This is because all new drugs are protected by patents which prevent other companies from making exact copies for several years after a drug is discovered. The medical effects of 'me-toos' are the same as those of the drugs they are

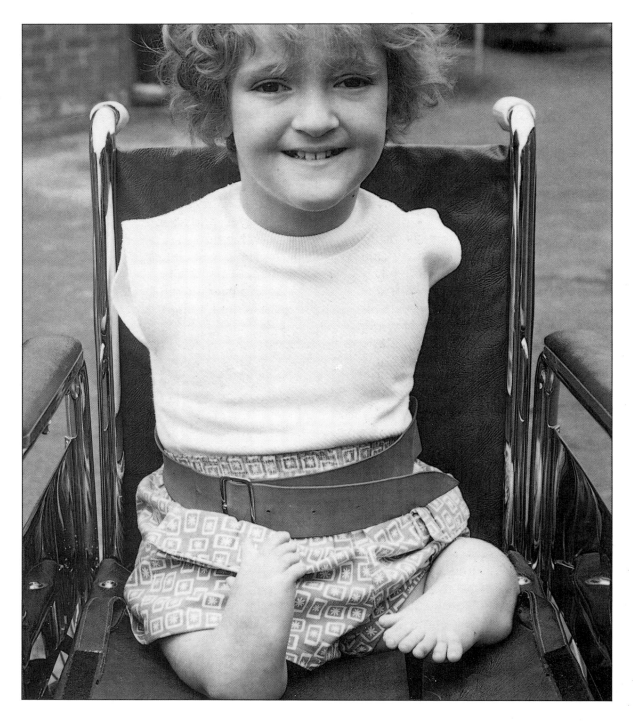

The thalodimide drug was given to pregnant women in the late 1950s. It was used as a sedative and helped prevent morning sickness. However, many of the babies were born with deformed limbs.

copying. The aim of the companies that make them is simply to take a slice of a very lucrative market.

Most 'me-toos' are for long-term illnesses. For example, there are literally dozens of very similar drugs for arthritis, high blood pressure, anxiety and sleep problems. Companies that make them point out small differences: slightly less side effects, slightly more effective in certain groups of patients, slightly easier to take.

Do these differences really justify so many 'me-toos' or should companies have spent the money looking for really important, new drugs? As we have already seen, it takes many years of research and many millions of pounds to find a really good new drug. And there are no guarantees of success. Drug companies argue that they need the profits from the drugs they are selling today – including 'me-toos' – to pay for future research. They insist that the small differences between 'me-toos' and their rivals are important to some patients. For example, it is well known that a patient with arthritis may stop responding to one drug and then feel much better with another very similar product. No one knows why this should be. But for the patient in pain it is important.

Clearly, it is not easy to judge whether drug companies should be allowed to spend their time making 'me-toos' instead of searching for life-saving drugs.

HARMFUL DRUGS

Thalidomide is not a name anyone is likely to forget. It was prescribed as a sedative to pregnant women in the late 1950s and many of their babies were born with seriously deformed limbs. It was thalidomide that had damaged them.

After the thalidomide tragedy, many countries introduced strict tests which all new drugs must pass before they can be sold. But, despite all the safety checks, some dangerous drugs have still become available.

In the early 1970s a drug called Eraldin was taken by thousands of people to control their blood pressure before doctors realized that it caused serious side effects to the eyes, and abdominal and connective tissues.

In 1982 the anti-arthritic drug, Opren, was banned in Britain because it was linked to liver and kidney problems. Some patients died. Others suffered long-term sensitivity to light. Their skin would blister or burn if they went out in the sun.

Yet, large numbers of people did benefit from Opren. Some doctors still believe the drug should be available for certain patients as long as they are carefully monitored.

Other drugs – for arthritis, depression and pain – have been banned or withdrawn in the years since the thalidomide tragedy.

The use of some drugs has been severely restricted because of side effects. A group of tranquillizers, of which Valium and Mogadon are best known, had been on the market for twenty years before official warnings went out about the problems of addiction. During that time millions of people had taken them – and suffered serious withdrawal problems when they tried to stop. Today, many thousands of people are still trying, some of them unsuccessfully, to give up their tranquillizers.

In 1991, one of this group of drugs, Halcion, was banned in Britain because of

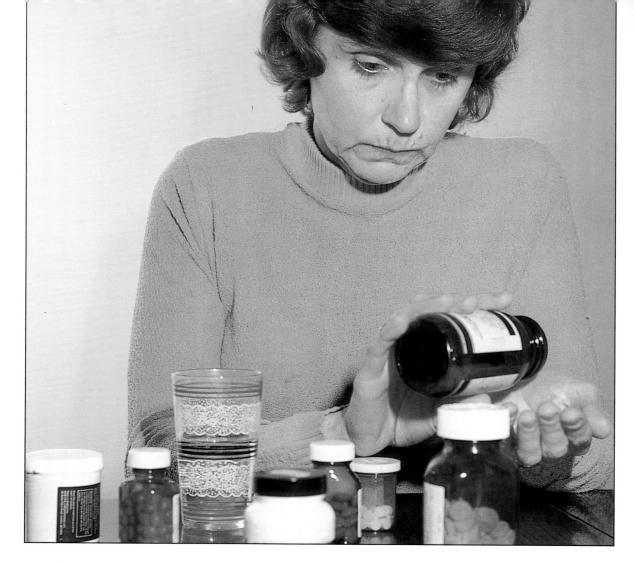

its side effects. It had taken doctors ten years to realise that the personality and memory disorders experienced by some people who took Halcion were so common that the risks of the drugs outweighed the benefits.

The story of this group of drugs, called benzodiazepines, is especially unfortunate. These drugs were brought in to replace a group of drugs called barbiturates which were, themselves, found to be addictive and were widely used to commit suicide. 'Benzos' were supposed to be the drugs the world had been waiting for. Sadly, the experts were wrong.

In the 1970s and 1980s many people became addicted to tranquillizers, which in some cases only made the original problem (usually depression) worse.

How is it that, despite all the experts and tests, such drugs can still cause so much trouble for the people who take them? What are the tests that drugs must pass before they can be sold and are such tests tough enough? Will it ever be possible to test new drugs so carefully that patients can be certain the treatment is safe?

CHAPTER FIVE

TESTING

FOR every drug that is sold as many as 10,000 fall by the wayside during the twelve years it takes to find and test a new product. Most will never even make it into the laboratory. But if a company is really unlucky its new drug can fall at the final hurdle – when it is being tested on humans – and many millions of pounds will be lost.

Much of the early design of new drugs is now done on computer screens. Scientists juggle chemical structures of possible new drugs until they have some likely candidates. They are looking for drugs that will compete with natural chemicals to fit the receptor sites in the body. Chemists then make these compounds and the tests begin.

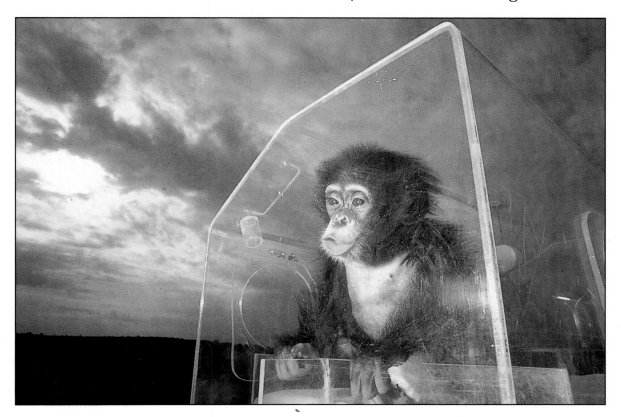

Using a chimp for medical research in a laboratory in New York. Many people think animal testing is cruel. However, few humans volunteer for testing and a drug cannot be released into the market unless it has been proved safe. Alternative methods for testing drugs are being sought.

Scientists test the new drug on small pieces of animal tissue. If these early tests work, the studies move to whole animals. Rats and mice are used most often. But rabbits, dogs and sometimes monkeys may also be needed.

At this stage the scientists are trying to find out not only if a drug works but also what side effects, if any, it has. Does it cause cancer, for example, if it is taken for long periods of time? And does it harm unborn animals if it is given to their pregnant mothers?

Scientists try to use fewer animals than they used to. Increasingly they can use clumps of cells, grown in the laboratory, to test drugs instead of whole animals. Rats and mice do not, after all, respond quite the same to drugs as humans and they do not have many of the same illnesses. So the results that are obtained from animal studies may not be a very good indicator of how humans will react to a new drug.

Drugs will continue to be tested on animals until other alternatives can be found. There are not many humans who would want to take a new drug that had not been tested.

Only when researchers are satisfied with the results of laboratory and animal tests do studies begin on humans. These can take a long time. Three-quarters of the time spent researching a new drug goes on human studies.

The first human tests are carried out on healthy volunteers. They are all carefully

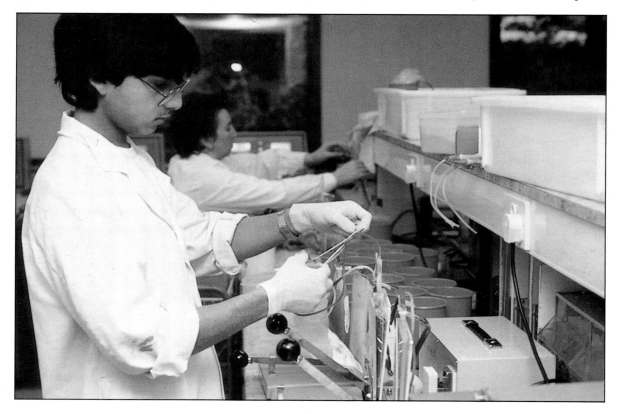

Testing drugs in a laboratory

watched after they have taken the drug. If, for example, a new blood pressure lowering drug is being tested, the volunteers' blood pressure is measured frequently and the volunteers are checked for any side effects.

The purpose of these early volunteer studies is also to get a better idea of the dose of a new drug that is needed.

When volunteer studies on twenty to thirty people are finished, trials begin on patients who are ill with the condition which the drug has been designed to treat. Before taking part in any studies they should be told all about the new drug and asked for their consent, in writing, to take part.

Patients are then divided into two groups. One group will be given the new drug and the other group will be given a dummy pill – or placebo. This is because some people feel better even when they are given an inactive drug and trials of a new product must take account of this. Researchers must be sure that any benefits they see with new drugs are genuine.

The patient studies gradually get larger and more complicated. There may be several groups of patients on different drugs, taking different doses.

By the time a company feels it has enough data to apply for a licence for a new drug, as many as 2000 people may have taken it in hospitals all over the world. They will have been examined and monitored every step of the way to ensure that the drug works and causes only minimal side effects.

The data from all the studies is then sent to an official licensing body. There is often enough data to fill a small room. An advisory committee of medical experts goes through all the data. It takes about a

year for the committee to assess all the information and decide whether to issue a licence. Only when a drug has a licence can it be put on the market.

Some drugs are licensed to be given to patients only when they are prescribed by a doctor while others can be bought in a chemist's shop. Some drugs can be sold, in small amounts, in shops and supermarkets, without the supervision of either a doctor or a pharmacist.

Research on a new drug does not stop once the drug is licensed. Studies continue

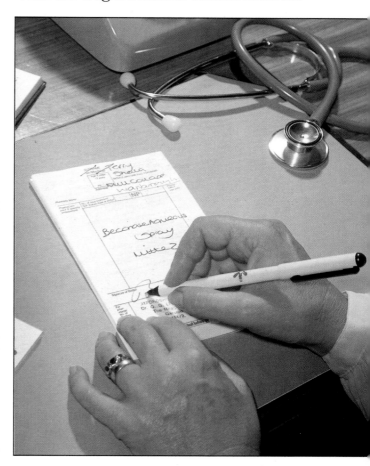

After numerous stringent tests, a new drug is issued a licence. It can then be prescribed by doctors.

long after it has come on to the market. Despite all the careful studies, the dose may turn out to be too high or too low for certain groups of patients. Great care will be taken in giving it to children, the elderly and women who are trying to get pregnant, since all these groups are vulnerable to problems.

The new drug is likely to be compared with its main rivals to see which is best. Doctors are asked to report any unusual side effects to the Committee on Safety of Medicines. That way, it is hoped that any problems will be detected early, before too many patients have taken the new drug. Serious side effects tend to be rare and it is only when many thousands of patients have taken a drug that they start to show up. Then the difficult decision must be made whether to restrict a drugs's use or ban it completely.

WHEN THINGS GO WRONG

When people are injured by drugs they have taken they may try to get compensation from the companies that made them. But this will probably take many years.

The amount of money they can expect will depend on how much damage the drug has caused. In some cases, companies have set up compensation funds. But, in other cases, victims have had to go to court with no guarantees of success.

The amount of money people are awarded also depends on where they go to court. In the USA, relatives of some

people who died after taking Opren received millions of dollars each in compensation – more than all the British victims put together.

Nowadays, people injured by drugs in Britain often try to take their cases through the US courts in the hope of getting more money, more quickly, especially if the drug they took was made by a US company. But the fact that courts in the USA make such large awards has had drawbacks too. Some companies have withdrawn useful drugs rather than risk expensive legal battles later on.

For example, in the USA it is no longer possible to get an intrauterine device (IUD) as a method of contraception. This followed a long legal battle involving an IUD manufacturer. Other companies decided not to risk keeping their IUDs on the market, though there was no substantial

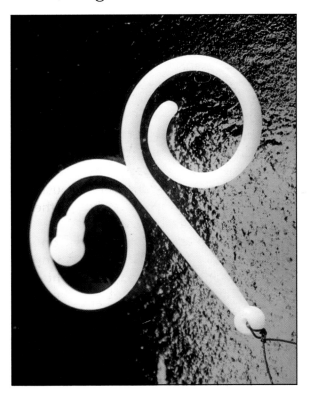

The controversial IUD (intrauterine) device has been banned as a method of contraception in the USA. This follows a major legal battle.

Drugs are a major business, especially in the USA where most medical care is private. Scandals are constantly being exposed.

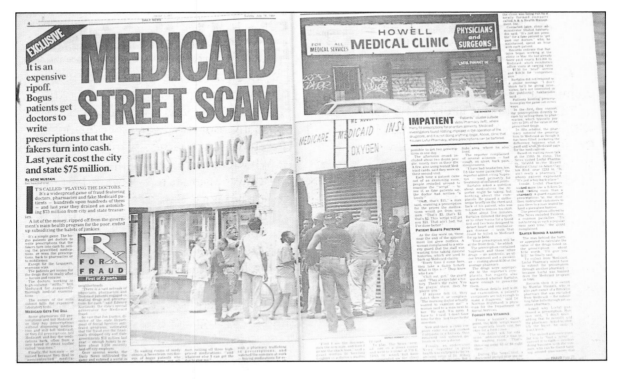

evidence against them. In Britain a number of IUDs are still available and many women are glad of the extra choice.

Companies can insure themselves against being sued over their drugs. But big compensation awards in the USA have also meant big increases in the insurance premiums that drug companies must pay. These extra costs are passed on to the consumer in higher priced drugs.

Until 1988 anyone injured by a drug in Britain had to prove that the company which made the drug was negligent – they had not taken enough care in testing or making the drug. This was almost impossible. Now, however, people in European Community (EC) countries only have to show that the drug caused their injuries. No cases have, as yet, come to

court under the new system. But it is hoped that it will make it easier for drug accident victims to get compensation.

Some experts believe that a compensation fund or an insurance scheme, similar to those in Sweden and New Zealand, would be fairer. People injured by drugs would get compensation without having to prove who was at fault. However, awards through such systems do tend to be smaller and, in New Zealand, the scheme ran into trouble because there was too little money for it.

Clearly, no one has yet found the best way to compensate people for drug accidents. We can only hope that, in the future, stricter testing will mean that fewer people will be damaged by drugs or need to seek compensation.

CHAPTER SIX

THE COST

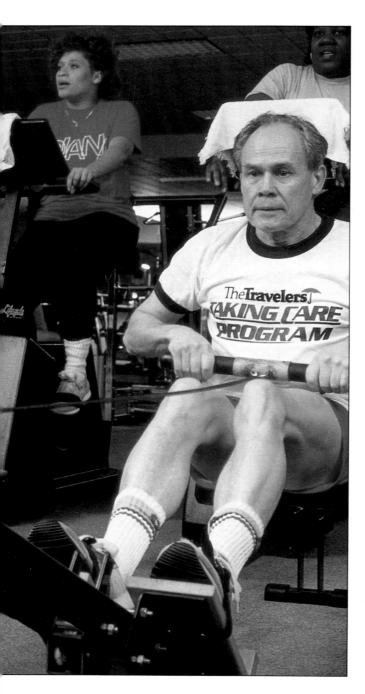

IT COSTS a drug company an estimated £150 million to discover and test a new drug and get it on to the market. Doctors already have some 4000 drugs to choose from but they only use about 200. So why do we need any more?

The answer is that there are more than enough drugs to treat some illnesses but too few to treat others. In Britain, doctors have restrictions about which drugs to prescribe. For example, they may choose from only a small number of tranquillizers.

Many hospitals have formularies: lists of drugs, drawn up by senior doctors, that may be used on the wards. Drugs not on the lists may only be used if there is a very good reason. Family doctors are also taking more account of the cost of the drugs they prescribe so that they can stay within their budgets.

Drug companies are being challenged to prove not only that their new drugs work and that they have few side effects but also that they are worth having. They are trying to show that people who take their drugs live longer and are less likely to need expensive hospital care when they get ill.

For example, someone who has too much cholesterol in their blood is more likely to have a heart attack. So a drug company that makes a drug which lowers cholesterol levels will argue that the cost

Medical experts are urging patients to take more responsibility for their health by eating healthily and exercising.

of taking the drug is well worth the saving in hospital bills because the patient is less likely to have a heart attack.

In planning future research, all companies are having to think much more carefully about how they will justify the price of their products. Unless they can prove the new drugs have real advantages over existing drugs, companies are going to find it harder and harder to get doctors to prescribe them.

Drug companies in Britain blame the government for reducing their profits and leaving them with less money to put into finding and testing new drugs. However, critics of the drug industry support the restrictions. They believe that companies will have to concentrate on looking for more real advances in medical treatment instead of producing more 'me-toos.'

PREVENTION IS BETTER THAN CURE

If a jumbo jet crashed every day, killing all its passengers, there would be an outcry. But that many people do indeed die every day from heart disease. Despite all the drugs and operations, heart disease kills over 120,000 people under seventy-five each year in Britain.

Most die because they smoked. Smoking kills around 100,000 people a year from lung and heart diseases. Others die because of a diet that contains too much fat, or because they were very overweight.

Most deaths from heart disease and lung cancer could be prevented. Someone who gives up smoking today will have lowered his or her risk of heart disease to that of a non-smoker within five years and the risk of lung cancer within ten to fifteen years.

Reducing the amount of cholesterol in your blood by just 10 per cent – by eating less fat – is thought to reduce the risk of heart disease by 20-30 per cent. Exercise is also important in reducing the risk of heart disease. It helps to keep weight

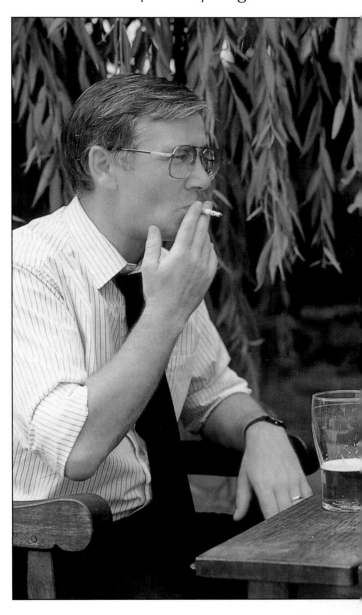

Cigarettes are one of the most dangerous drugs, causing the deaths of about 100,000 people a year in Britain.

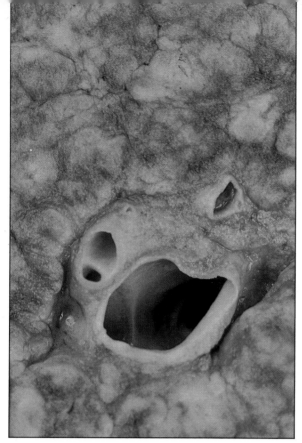

A close-up of a liver specimen showing cirrhosis caused by alcohol.

there was a 40 per cent drop. But in England and Wales deaths fell by only 11 per cent.

The British Government set a target for the year 2000. It wants to see a 30 per cent reduction in heart disease deaths among people under sixty-five and a drop in the number of people who smoke from 32 per cent to 21 per cent. There must also be big reductions in the amount of fat consumed.

This can be achieved by having a diet that contains less red and fatty meat and more chicken and fish. It should also have less butter, cream and other dairy products and fewer processed foods like biscuits and cake. Instead, people should try to eat more fresh fruit and vegetables.

If this is to succeed, we need to start young. Children who are overweight or who do not take enough exercise turn into fat adults with high blood pressure and a high risk of heart disease.

down and has a beneficial effect on the balance of fats in the blood.

In contrast, lowering blood pressure (the other main risk factor for heart disease) with drugs, reduces the risk of a heart attack by less than 15 per cent.

So why do we not change our diet and life-style instead of relying on expensive drugs, which may have side effects, when we become ill? Doctors have pondered this question for many years. Despite all the warnings, we continue to smoke, eat unwisely and take too little exercise.

Some countries have heeded the warnings. In the USA many people have changed to a more healthy life-style. Between 1970 and 1985 the number of people who died from heart disease fell by 50 per cent. In Australia, Israel and Canada

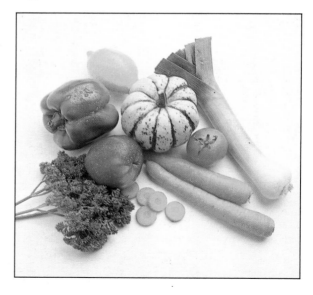

Heart disease can often be prevented by keeping to a healthy diet of fresh fruit and vegetables.

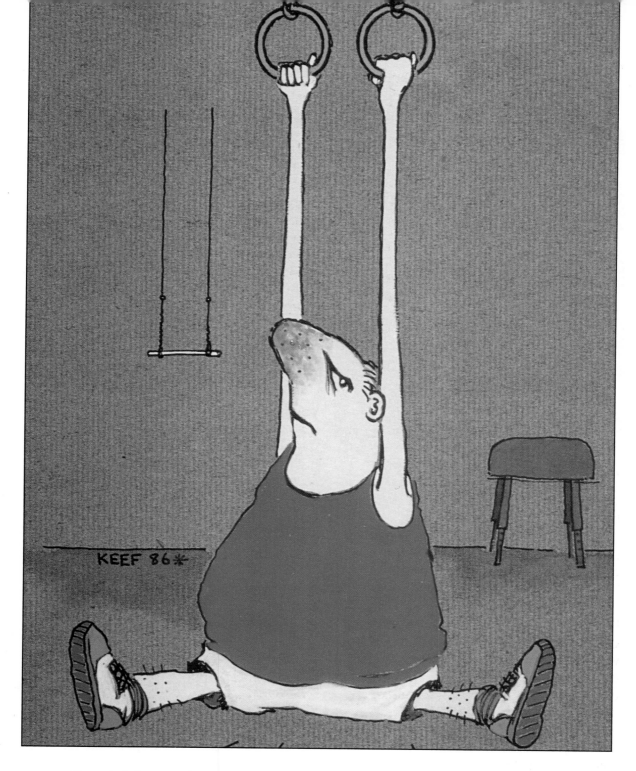

Overweight people are more at risk of suffering heart disease and high blood pressure. Exercise is being promoted as a way of preventing potentially fatal illnesses.

CHAPTER SEVEN

HOMEOPATHY AND HERBALISM

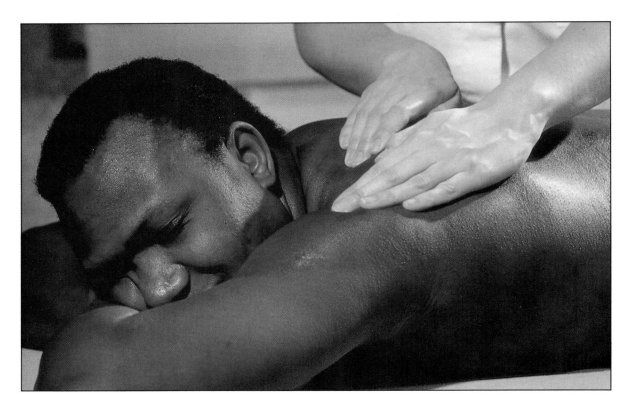

IN RECENT years, many people have become dissatisfied with the type of medicine that most doctors practise. Some are worried about the side effects of modern drugs. They feel that the risks outweigh the benefits. They have tried to find gentler ways of helping the body to overcome illness.

Homeopathy uses natural remedies to treat the whole person, not just his or her symptoms. People who practise homeopathy (homeopaths) believe that symptoms such as headache, fever and sickness are the body's way of fighting illness. So they use very small amounts of natural substances which, if they were used in larger quantities, would actually cause symptoms.

Homeopaths believe that the more closely a remedy imitates patients' symptoms the more likely it is to heal them. Also, the more dilute it is, the better. This means that, often, the active ingredients of a homeopathic remedy are undetectable in the liquid they have been dissolved in.

Doctors who practise conventional medicine find it hard to accept that such remedies can work. In general, the stronger a drug used in orthodox

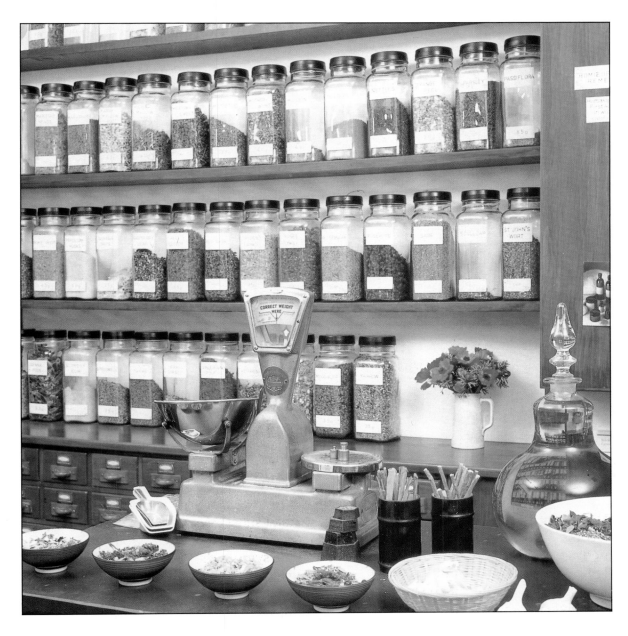

OPPOSITE **This man is being given an aromatherapy massage. In aromatherapy, fragrant herb and flower extracts, known as essential oils, are massaged into the skin. Alternatively, they can be inhaled or put into creams or lotions. Different fragrances are used for different problems or symptoms.**

ABOVE **Shelves containing jars of dried flowers and plants in a herbal dispensary. Herbal medicine has been practised by many cultures for thousands of years and has gained limited acceptance by the medical profession. Herbal medicines can be taken as capsules or hot water infusions.**

medicine, the better it works. Homeo-pathic treatment has been hard to test scientifically because it usually includes many different remedies. But the fact that so many people pay for homeopathic treatment suggests that they believe they are benefitting.

The same is true of herbal remedies. Doctors who practise conventional medicine are more wary of them as they are more likely to cause side effects than homeopathic treatments. This is because larger amounts are used.

A lot of modern medicines are derived from plants and herbs and many drug companies are studying plants to see if more drugs can be obtained from them. However, just because a product is 'natural' does not mean it is safe. Many plants and herbs are poisonous and they should be used only by people who understand what is in them and how they work.

Like homeopathic treatment, very few herbal remedies have been tested scientifically. Notable exceptions include evening primrose oil which is used in a wide range of conditions from arthritis to menstrual problems, and feverfew which is used to treat migraines.

The general lack of studies is a major obstacle to homeopathic and herbal remedies being accepted by most doctors who practice conventional medicine. As we have already seen, doctors rely on the results of studies of new drugs to decide whether to use them. They need evidence to back up the claims of drug firms and, in the case of homeopathic and herbal medicine, there is very little.

More effort is being made to test some of these products and, hopefully, this will at last help to clear up some of the doubts. It seems clear that homeopathy and herbalism are going to assume more popularity and importance in the future.

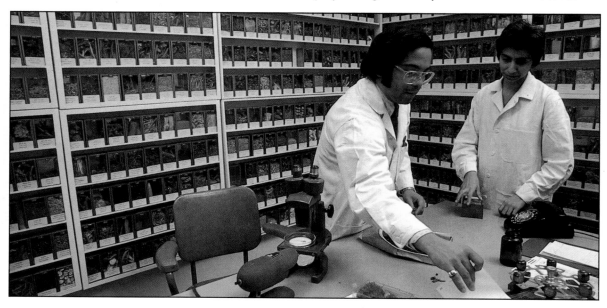

A herb library in New Jersey, USA which stores all the herb and plant types that can be used in herbalism.

CHAPTER EIGHT

WHAT DO WE WANT ?

IN 1990 British doctors wrote 446 million prescriptions for drugs. That is eight prescriptions a year for every man, woman and child. The number is steadily increasing all the time.

One reason that doctors are prescribing more drugs is that the population is getting older and therefore more likely to be ill. Many of us have come to rely on drugs to make us feel better when perhaps we do not need really need them.

Many doctors are not very good at saying 'no'! It is much quicker and easier for a doctor to write a prescription than it is to explain what is actually wrong with us and that a drug might not be necessary. When the waiting room is full of patients, the doctor is likely to take the easy option and simply scribble out a prescription.

Does it really matter? Yes, it does! Not only are unnecessary drugs a waste of money but they may cause harm. Even

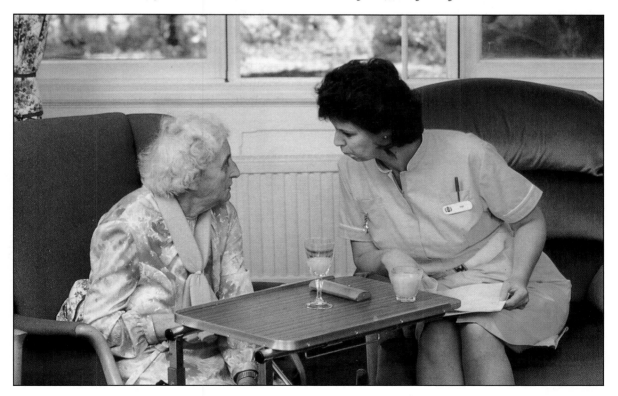

Many old people suffer from some form of dementia - a degeneration of the brain tissue. Symptoms include memory disorders, changes in personality and confusion. The cause is unknown and as yet there is no cure.

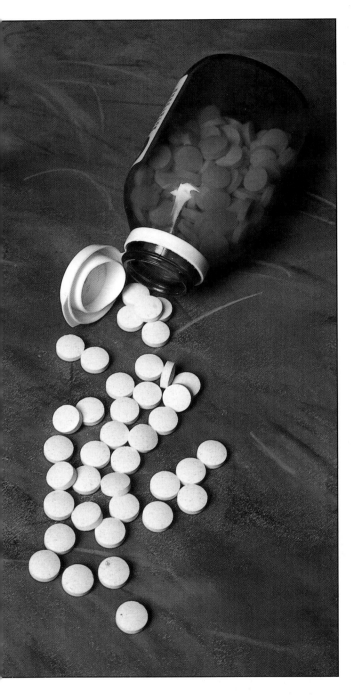

Many people take drugs unnecessarily. Illnesses, such as the common cold and some stomach upsets can be treated at home without the use of pills.

drugs for minor ailments have side effects. For example, some decongestants used to unblock stuffy noses should not be used by people with high blood pressure or who are taking a particular type of antidepressant drug.

Aspirin and aspirin-like drugs can make some people's stomachs bleed, especially the elderly, and should not be taken if they are not really needed. There are many varieities of this type of drug available on the market. People often buy the pills without being fully aware of what they are.

There is no cure for the common cold, which is caused by a virus. Yet many people are prescribed antibiotics which work against bacteria, not against viruses. So, not only are the drugs ineffective against the cold, they may disturb the natural balance of microbes in our body and, when they are used against a bacterial infection, they may not work.

Many people take unnecessary drugs, including antibiotics, for stomach upsets. The best treatment for an upset stomach is to stop eating, and take plenty of liquids, with sugar and salt if you are very dehydrated, to replace those lost by diarrhoea and vomiting. Then wait for the body's own defence cells to get rid of the infection. Taking drugs to stop the diarrhoea may prolong the attack. Drugs are rarely needed unless the upset goes on for a week or more.

There is a lot we can do for ourselves when we are ill. Reaching for a pill bottle or rushing to the doctor for minor coughs, colds and stomach upsets is not always the answer.

When we go to the doctor we should not always expect a prescription for drugs. A little reassurance that there is nothing seriously wrong is often all that is needed.

Doctors' time could be used more effectively. Rather than always asking for another prescription for another bottle of pills, patients could take more responsibility for their own health by discussing the problems with doctors.

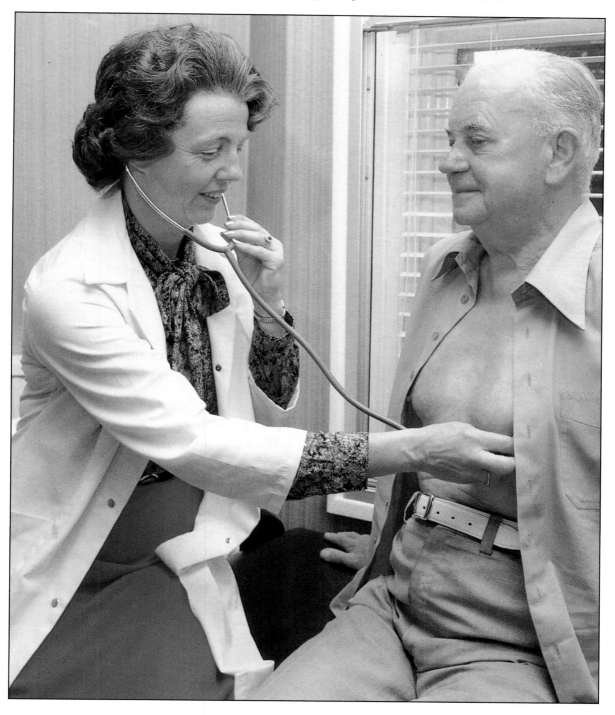

CHAPTER NINE

FUTURE CURES

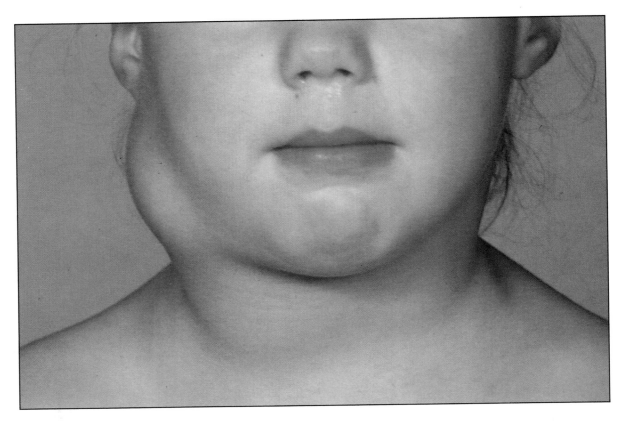

CANCER, dementia, AIDS, Parkinson's disease, muscle wasting disorders, strokes and heart attacks are just a few of today's diseases still awaiting cures.

Cancer treatment has improved a lot in the last twenty years. Some childhood cancers, testicular cancer and Hodgkin's disease – cancer of the lymph glands – have high cure rates, thanks largely to better anti-cancer drugs.

Recently, it has been shown that women with early breast cancer do a lot better if they have anti-cancer drugs after surgery to remove their tumour.

But little progress has been made with the biggest killer, lung cancer. Overall, only about half of people who get cancer survive it.

Future advances in cancer treatment are likely to come through genetic screening. Doctors hope to detect people who are at high risk of cancer because of abnormal genes so they can be treated much earlier, before the tumour has a chance to spread.

Dementia is probably the greatest challenge to medical scientists. Very little is known about what causes it. So the chances of a cure in the near future are

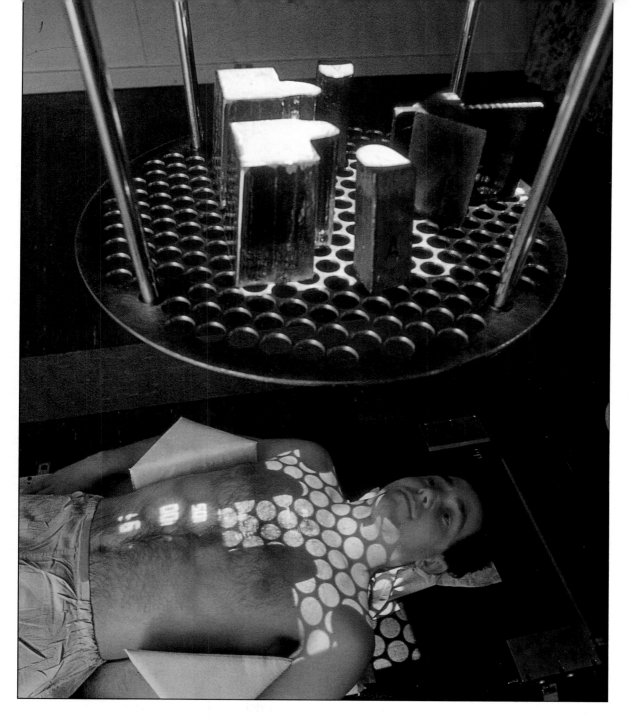

OPPOSITE **A child suffering from Hodgkin's disease - a cancer of the lymphatic system. Treatment depends on the extent of the disease and may include surgery, radiotherapy and chemotherapy, or a combination of all three.**

ABOVE **A patient undergoing radiotherapy to treat Hodgkin's disease. The illuminated discs over his chest show which areas are to receive radiation, thus protecting the lungs from excessive irradiation.**

remote. Yet, with our ageing population, it is vital that a breakthrough comes soon.

We know the nerves in the brains of people with dementia become tangled. Some people with dementia have a gene defect. And dementia is more common among people with a high aluminium intake. But what does it all add up to? No one is sure.

The outlook for people with AIDS is better. A lot of progress has been made in developing drugs for the disease since it was first recognized in the early 1980s. People with AIDS live longer now. There are drugs which attack the AIDS virus and there is better treatment for the serious infections that people with AIDS suffer from because of their damaged immune systems.

But no one is pretending that we are near to a cure for AIDS and it will be difficult to develop an effective vaccine because the AIDS virus is changing. So it is very important that we all continue to take steps to prevent the spread of AIDS by avoiding unsafe sexual contact, drug abuse or infected blood.

Current drugs for Parkinson's disease can treat symptoms in the early stages. But gradually the drugs stop working so well and patients lose control over their ability to move and speak. Some progress has been made in understanding why the nerves in the brain become damaged but there is still a long way to go before drugs are available to stop or even reverse the damage.

Doctors are very interested in a new group of drugs, called anti-oxidants, which may have widespread uses in many of today's common diseases, including strokes, heart attacks, Parkinson's disease and arthritis.

In the last few years, scientists have begun to realize that many of the normal metabolic reactions in the cells have adverse effects. They produce by-products called oxygen radicals which damage tissues. For example, they interact with the molecules that make up the membranes of cells. So the membranes break down and the cells die. This sort of process occurs following strokes and heart attacks.

Luckily, scientists have discovered some 'anti-oxidants' which stop the oxygen radicals from being formed and prevent cells from being destroyed. These are now being tested in a great number of diseases.

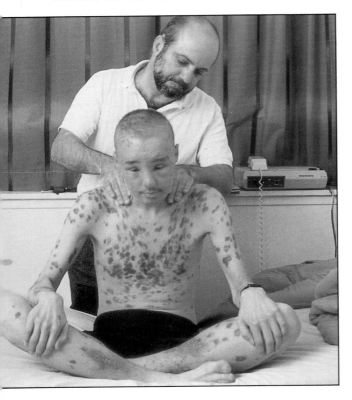

An AIDS patient being treated by a nurse. The AIDS virus damages the immune system so sufferers are prone to serious infections.

This false-colour scanning electron micrograph (SEM) shows a killer cell (green) attacking a large cancer tumour cell (pink and yelow). The killer cell, a white blood cell, must make contact with the tumour cell in order to destroy it. The tumour cell may survive, however, by budding off blisters (seen here) which form a protective barrier between itself and the killer cell.

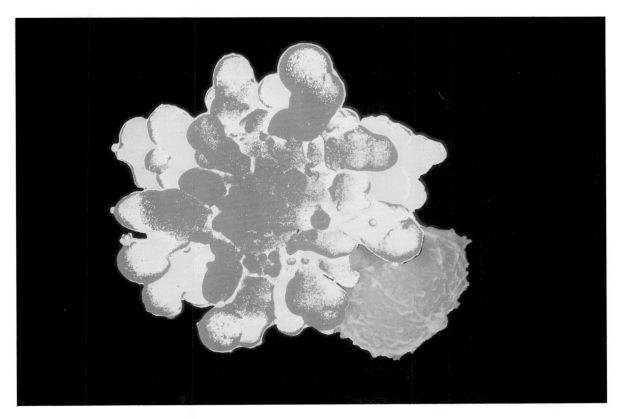

Sadly, little progress has been made in the treatment of muscle wasting disorders, such as Duchenne muscular dystrophy. But doctors can now test a foetus in the womb for the faulty gene responsible for the disease. If a baby is likely to be affected its parents can be given the choice of having the pregnancy terminated.

Genetic testing may well hold the key to preventing and, ultimately, treating many of today's incurable diseases. A massive international research project is underway to map all the genes on the twenty-three pairs of human chromosomes. It is likely to take many years. Hopefully, when the map is complete, doctors will know much more about the genetic abnormalities that make us prone to physical illnesses, including cancer and heart disease and mental disorders, such as depression, schizophrenia and dementia. They may, in the future, even be able to replace abnormal genes with normal ones. The first attempts at gene therapy have already been made and the early results are promising.

GLOSSARY

Antibody A defence protein that protects the body from invading micro-organisms and other substances.

Bacterium A type of micro-organism which causes infections, such as tuberculosis, whooping cough, and most cases of food poisoning.

Dementia The progressive and ultimately fatal deterioration in mental ability which occurs mainly in elderly people.

Enzyme The substance needed for a chemical reaction to occur.

Gene The basic unit found on chromosomes in the centre of every cell which determines a person's physical and mental characteristics.

Genetic engineering Changes to or movement of genes, carried out in the laboratory to alter the structure or function of a cell or organism.

Hormone A chemical which is made in one part of the body but has an effect in a different part.

Inflammation Painful reddening or swelling.

IUD Intrauterine contraceptive device, which is put into a woman's womb to prevent an embryo from attaching itself to the wall of the womb. It probably also stops sperm travelling up through the womb to fertilize an egg.

Membrane The outer layer of a cell which keeps most of the contents inside but allows some chemicals to pass in and out.

Menopause The time in a woman's life after which she can no longer have children, owing to a fall in her female hormones. Usually occurs around the age of fifty.

Metabolism The chemical processes that occur within a living organism.

Micro-organism An organism, such as a bacterium or virus, which can only be seen through a microscope.

Multiple sclerosis A nerve disorder in which nerves lose their outer coating so they can no longer carry messages to the tissues, leading eventually to paralysis and death. But the disease is unpredictable and people can live a long time without getting any worse.

Nerve transmitter A chemical needed to carry messages from one nerve to another.

Vaccine A substance which is injected into the body to make it produce protective antibodies against infectious organisms.

Virus A micro-organism, much smaller than a bacterium, that causes infections such as chickenpox, colds and flu.

FURTHER READING

Diet and Health by Ida Weekes (Wayland, 1991)
Disease and Discovery by Eva Bailey (Batsford, 1987)
Drugs by Christian Wolmar (Wayland, 1990)
Drugs and Crime by Marcella Foster and Joe Sheehan (Wayland, 1992)
Drugs and Sport by Christian Wolmar (Wayland, 1992)
Drugs and the Media by Scarlett MccGwire (Wayland, 1992)
Health and Medicine by Brenda Walpole (Wayland, 1990)
Let's Discuss Aids by Graham Wilkinson (Wayland, 1987)
Let's Discuss Health and Fitness by Tony Wheatley (Wayland, 1988)
Medical Ethics by Jenny Bryan (Wayland, 1989)
Smoking by Anne Charlish (Wayland, 1990)
The Body and How it Works by Steve Barker (Dorling Kindersley, 1987)
The Human Body by Ruth and Bertel Bruun (Kingfisher Books, 1985)
Twentieth Century Medicine by Jenny Bryan (Wayland, 1988)

ACKNOWLEDGEMENTS

Camera Press 28 (Geoff Howard); Colorific 4 (Jim Pickerell), 8 (Jean Claude Lejeune), 27 (Mitchell Funk Wheeler Pictures), 38 (Martin Rogers), 44 (Alan Reininger); Department of Medical Illustration/St Bartholomew's Hospital 34 (top); Jeff Greenberg 16, 31; National Medical Slide Bank 14, 23, 35, 39, 42; Science Photo Library COVER (Tim Beddow), (Adam Hart-Davis),7 (CNRI), 9 (Jim Selby), 10 (Andrew McClenaghan), 6, Bill Longcore, 11, David Gifford, 12, 13 (Alexander Tsiaris), 15 (Dr Beer-Gabel/CNRI), 17 (Simon Fraser), 22 (top, David Leah, bottom, National Institute of Health), 26, 27, (Shelia Terry) 32 (Hank Morgan), 33 (Adam Hart-Davis), 36 (Damien Lovegrove), 37 (Paul Biddle), 43 (Martin Dohrn), 47 (Dr Andrejs Liepins); Tony Stone Worldwide 5; Topham Picture Library 16, 40; Wayland Picture Library 24, 34 (bottom), 41.

INDEX

This book is to be returned on or before
the last date stamped below.